I0504129

The Logical Basis of Clinical Medicine by Mark S. Rosenberg.
First Edition © 2013. Second Edition © 2019. All rights reserved.

Group purchase rates are available.

Address correspondence to: Logical Arts Press, 4 South Pomperaug Avenue, Woodbury, CT 06798 or L.A.PRESS8@gmail.com

Available on amazon.com

MARK S. ROSENBERG, MD

THE

LOGICAL BASIS OF

CLINICAL MEDICINE

An Introduction to Diagnosis-Driven Analysis
in Clinical Practice

CONTENTS

PREFACE
To the Second Edition

It has been six years since the first edition of this book was published. The impetus for this second edition is to correct some typographical errors and edit specific sections in order to express certain ideas more clearly.

The fundamental concepts discussed have not changed.

This is a book about something physicians use all the time in clinical medicine: the diagnosis.

The primary act in treating a patient who is ill is to create a relationship between the disease in the patient and its corresponding diagnosis. It is worthwhile, therefore, to understand exactly what a diagnosis is and how it comes into being.

The most important thing a diagnosis provides is a context by which to interpret our observations of disease. Likewise, a patient's medical history, comprised of all the diagnoses that a patient carries, provides a context by which to understand and treat the patient.

While the substantive ideas in this book have not changed, clinical medicine has evolved dramatically since this book was first published. For one, the electronic medical record (EMR) has become the predominant, if not the exclusive, repository of clinical information.

The diagnosis is a symbolic representation of the logical form of the disease with which it is associated. A diagnosis is created by treating the signs of disease as symbolic elements and relating them to one another in a manner that is consistent with their behavior in the real world.

In the same way, the EMR holds a symbolic representation of clinical activity. For the EMR to work, it must work on a conceptual level. It must provide, by way of analogy, a representation of the logical form of clinical activity.

The reader will find that many of the ideas presented in this book provide insight into how an EMR needs to be structured if it is to accomplish this goal.

While the subject of this book is the concept of the diagnosis and its relationship to the logical form of disease, its objective more generally is to promote clear and coherent thinking in clinical medicine.

By learning principles of symbolic logic and applying them to the practice of clinical medicine, it is hoped that physicians, as well as others involved in the field of health care, can acquire the conceptual tools necessary to analyze the problems which they find in clinical medicine and be guided in the direction of effective solutions.

M. S. Rosenberg, M.D.
October 2019

PROLOGUE

This book is a highly focused introduction to the essentials of logical structure specifically as they relate to clinical medicine.

Each chapter has been designed to build upon that which precedes it. It is important, particularly if these ideas are difficult for the reader to understand or are forcing the reader to think in a manner he or she is not naturally inclined, to give some time to contemplate the ideas presented in one chapter before moving on to the next; otherwise, the discussion may seem to be aimless and unsystematic.

All physicians receive training in bedside clinical skills, diagnostics, and decision-making. The ideas discussed here are not intended to replace such training; nor should it be inferred from the ideas presented in this book that these approaches are somehow lacking. The topics discussed here are primarily conceptual and, if anything, might serve to supplement such clinical training.

There is no attempt here to discuss developments in the field of decision analysis and other analytic strategies that have been applied to clinical work; such a discussion is unnecessary and would add very little except for additional length.

When the word "sign" is employed in this book, it is often used in its logical sense and not in the manner in which physicians most often use the term, which is to indicate physical stigmata of disease.

The illustrations that accompany the text are intended to provide graphic representations of the ideas being discussed. Some of these concepts can be better understood when presented in pictorial format, as opposed to the discursive presentation that language requires.

To some readers, these ideas may seem more philosophical than clinical, and perhaps even a play in the world of semantics as opposed to discussing any substantive issues relevant to clinical medicine. To some, the information contained in these chapters may seem to be mere opinion. In fact, these ideas represent a body of knowledge that is primarily mathematical in nature. Doctors in clinical practice deal with clinical data. Mathematicians deal with concepts. Doctors try to relate clinical facts to each other. Mathematicians try to relate concepts to each other.

In many instances, the concepts with which mathematicians work have application in the real world; the attempt here is to show how concepts of logical structure relate to clinical medicine.

The specific knowledge that the physician is intended to gain is of the essentials of logical structure and how it applies to clinical medicine. While there is no guarantee that these ideas will improve the care of individual patients or render clinical activity more satisfying to the doctor, some might find these ideas interesting and others may find they promote habits of clear and coherent thought and, in so doing, yield the potential to improve the analysis of their patients' medical conditions and communication with other health care providers about clinical matters.

Throughout this book, wherever the word doctor or physician is used, one can substitute, without a significant change in meaning, the terms "medical assistant," "nurse," "physician assistant," "health care provider," or indeed the designation of any individual whose job requires him or her to recognize the presence of disease.

M. S. Rosenberg, M.D.
July 2013

Dedicated to *Sir Isaac Newton* and *Albert Einstein*, individuals who studied nature in search of logical form.

To arrive at the simplest truth, as Newton knew and practiced, requires *years of contemplation*. Not activity. Not reasoning. Not calculating. Not busy behavior of any kind. Not reading. Not talking. Not making an effort. Not thinking. Simply *bearing in mind* what it is one needs to know.

- G. Spencer-Brown, *mathematician*

Everything should be made as simple as possible, but not simpler.

- Albert Einstein, *physicist*

Chapter One
Clinical Medicine and Symbolic Logic

1.1 A New Age of Medicine and Its Conceptual Tools

We have entered a new age of medicine. The transition did not come all at once, in one fell swoop, leaving traditional medicine behind and introducing a new age which lies ahead of us. It has been ushered in slowly and hesitantly.

The signs of the new age are clear, however. The electronic medical record is but one such sign. Hand-held electronic devices, streaming clinical information to the physician continually, are another. The ability to extract clinical data in a wide range of forms and formats, in a wide range of locations, and toward a wide range of purposes is now commonplace.

Yet the conceptual tools at physicians' disposal remain largely the same. We continue to talk to each other about patients. We write notes in charts. Some of us may type notes in charts. We dictate. Perhaps the newest addition to our armamentarium is when we point and click on a computer screen to enter clinical data; but even still, the movements are ultimately transformed into letters and numbers, words and sentences, perhaps pictures, and eventually reports.

And the clinical data is stored, somehow, somewhere, in bits and pieces, here and there, to appear at some time, in various ways, so we can keep track of it all and take care of our patients.

The clinical data originates, in the beginning and always, from the patient. The history is taken. A physical exam is performed. Laboratory data is reviewed. Radiology, now such a quaint and perhaps outdated term, provides all sorts of images. And the doctor studies the data. And interprets it. And establishes a diagnosis.

The process is so intuitive to the seasoned clinician that most physicians are largely unconscious of any system they utilize to make the leap from the sense-data derived from the evaluation of the patient to the construction of ideas and concepts about the patient's medical condition; ideas which the doctor creates and are needed in order to manage the patient.

It might seem odd to think that there exists a mathematical system that the physician uses to establish a diagnosis. The system certainly wasn't built for that purpose. It is perhaps more correct to say that there exists a mathematical system, created without medicine in mind, that informs us about what a physician does when he or she makes that leap from the patient to establish a diagnosis.

That system is called *symbolic logic.*

1.2 **Trouble in Paradise**
Why should we bother to learn about such a system, if we can already do our work without it?

Because there is trouble in paradise. And the symptoms are becoming increasingly apparent. We receive reports from the Emergency Department utilizing generic descriptors to describe all patients who present with pain of any sort. Colleagues send us office notes totaling 5 or 6 pages or more comprised primarily of generic text meant to describe the specifics of a particular patient's medical situation. And discharge summaries from the local hospital not uncommonly describe the hospital course of a patient by issues organized primarily into various specialties of medicine, as opposed to diagnoses, so that a patient presenting with an irregular heart rhythm, slurred speech, and weakness in one limb, is described, first and foremost, in terms of "cardiac" and "neuro" issues and only secondarily as a patient with atrial fibrillation who had a cerebral vascular accident.

The recipient of such reports, who might read them, but is perhaps without the benefit of having interviewed and examined the patient, not infrequently is left wondering: what actually happened with this patient? The desire to standardize our approach to the patient and generalize about an individual patient's specific presentation results in a report that seems to lose something in the translation.

1.3 **Generalization in Clinical Medicine**

The clinician must move from the consideration of a specific instance of a patient's presentation to more general concepts about a particular patient's medical condition. That is the only way in which a treatment plan can be devised. It is the only way a doctor may have some assurance that a treatment plan stands a chance of working.

Although doctors identify symptoms and physical stigmata of a disease, they do not really see the disease as an actual object, as one would see a house or a chair.

If doctors did not generalize about symptoms and physical stigmata of disease and attribute to them a hypothetical, purely reasoned history of causes, as well as a future of possible consequences, they could not recognize the symptoms and physical stigmata as a disease in the first place.

3

But all generalization is not equally effective.

For instance, to formulate a paragraph on a patient, whose electrocardiogram shows atrial fibrillation, with the general heading, "cardiac," and, in the next paragraph, start with the heading or generalization, "neuro," because the same patient also has neurological deficits, does not necessarily indicate any relationship between the "cardiac" and the "neuro" problems that the patient has, although they may, in fact, be related.

There are many diseases that can be classified as "cardiac" that have no relationship to diseases that are classified as "neuro." While the reader of the report will see these two general ideas first, as paragraph headings, neither contributes to the clinician's understanding of the patient in a particularly meaningful manner. Moreover, all patients with both cardiac and neurological issues, who are presented in this manner, will superficially appear similar, at least in the report, although in reality their medical conditions may be significantly different.

It would be more productive to compose one paragraph under the general heading "atrial fibrillation" (instead of "cardiac") and the other with the heading "cerebral vascular accident" (instead of ""neuro"). To say that the patient has "atrial fibrillation" brings to mind a whole host of causes and consequences. While data, such as the abnormal electrocardiogram, provides a clinical fact, *it is the general concept of a disease that gives that fact meaning*.

Likewise, it is much more productive to generalize about a patient's slurred speech and limb weakness by calling it a cerebral vascular accident, because it provides a more effective scheme for the clinician to understand the patient's presentation in terms of its supposed causes and future consequences.

But perhaps most important, only by generalizing and calling one abnormality atrial fibrillation and the other a cerebral vascular accident does the doctor draw a possible relationship between the two and thereby formulate a treatment plan that might treat one and reduce the risk of the other occurring again.

Since generalization is the business of logic, it would appear that the possibility for a productive partnership of clinical medicine and logic exists. Logic deals only with the general form of a thing, and not a specific instance of that thing.

The application of logic to clinical medicine leads one to understand the importance of *"diagnosis-driven" medicine* – a concept that will be further developed in Chapter 4. One of the goals of the clinician is to develop the "diagnostic personality" of each patient.

1.4 **Specialty Medicine and Communication**

Communication between and among physicians is becoming of paramount importance these days as the clinical practice of medicine is splintered into diverse and disparate functional groups. The broad clinical arenas of medicine and surgery, distinguished by conceptual and technical areas of expertise, have given forth to a wide range of subspecialties, including, for example, rheumatology, dermatology, cardiology, cardiothoracic surgery, colo-rectal surgery, and orthopedics. These, in turn, have given rise to physicians with expertise in a number of sub-subspecialties, such as non-invasive and interventional cardiology.

Most recently there has been specialization based not primarily on or exclusively due to conceptual or technical requirements, but, at least in part, due to economic necessity.

Many primary care physicians, fully capable intellectually, and equipped with all the conceptual skills and knowledge required to provide competent care to their hospitalized patients, those patients followed in the office but whose conditions require that they transition from the realm of outpatient medicine into the inpatient, hospital arena, where acute care needs to be rendered, now frequently delegate such activity to another group of physicians, the hospitalists, in part because of financial considerations.

While this is a perfectly legitimate practice pattern to follow, for those physicians who choose to do so, as the profitability of a service is a signal of its real or perceived value in the marketplace, it does raise a number of issues that should be considered.

For one, delegation of such inpatient clinical work to others has the potential to lead to a lapse in communication, *an information gap*, which can be highly problematic for optimal patient care.

1.5 The Observation of Disease and Interpretation

When primary care physicians follow their patients exclusively in the outpatient or office setting, and delegate the care of patients to the hospitalist for inpatient services, they are no longer privy to the observations of disease in all its manifestations across the entire spectrum of its history.

Those primary care physicians who use hospitalists exclusively, therefore, rely on the observations of these fellow physicians to tell them something about the acute phase of an illness in a patient who requires inpatient evaluation, because the primary care physicians no longer have the opportunity or perhaps even the privilege of observing this phase of the disease personally and directly.

So, too, the hospitalist does not see the full spectrum of a disease, because that doctor has no first-hand, direct exposure to the disease process as it unfolds in the outpatient arena. The best the hospitalist can hope for is information obtained through various reports from and conversations with those physicians who have cared for the patient in the outpatient setting.

A similar situation holds for many other physicians, who find themselves in the position of referring the care of a patient, in total and for a limited period of time, to some other physician, perhaps because of the need for highly specialized care or because the service the patient requires must be delivered in a place of service to which the referring physician has no access.

All clinicians understand, however, that the direct observation of symptoms and physical stigmata of disease must form the basis of our ideas and concepts about disease. The validity of such sense-knowledge is difficult to contradict and is the starting point for establishing diagnoses. It is the origin of evidence-based medicine. Sense-data, such as the symptoms felt by the patient, the direct observation of physical stigmata of disease, the personal perusal of all the laboratory data, the review of the pertinent diagnostic imaging with the radiologist, are the facts upon which our diagnostic constructs are based.

As clinicians grow away from that ideal of observing these so-called facts of disease first-hand, they rely more and more on other clinicians' interpretations of these facts. In so doing, clinicians are left in a position where they must take another clinician's *interpretation* of symptoms and physical stigmata of the disease with which the patient presents *as fact.*

The *process of interpretation* in clinical medicine, therefore, becomes exceptionally important to all clinicians who work together collaboratively. Equally important is the ability to communicate our interpretations and their implications in terms of the evaluation and treatment of a patient to other clinicians in the most concise, articulate manner.

1.6 Logic, Math, and Medicine
Most physicians use logic to construct their interpretations of the sense-data about disease. For example, if a patient with a fifty pack-year history of tobacco consumption presents with dyspnea on exertion and has a pulmonary function test that shows a severe obstructive pattern, a diagnosis of chronic obstructive pulmonary disease is established and appropriate treatment can be prescribed. But few physicians understand the principles of logic in any formal sense and how they are applied in this situation.

Logic is a branch of mathematics. The marriage between math and medicine is nothing new and the history of medicine is replete with a rapprochement between these two fields of study. The interpretation of signs of disease, for instance, is predicated on knowledge of mathematical constructs such as the *sensitivity, specificity, positive predictive value,* and *negative predictive value* of those signs. Clinical studies frequently employ the *p test,* a mathematical concept originating in the field of statistics, to test for the differences between two groups in order to reach conclusions, for example, about the efficacy of some particular treatment.

But there has been little formal analysis in medicine about how and why a collection of patients might be considered to form a distinct group in the first place. Logic is a branch of mathematics that speaks to this subject and informs us of the principles underlying the process by which such distinctions are made.

This book will serve to introduce the clinician to the essential features of logical structure[1] and how they relate to clinical medicine. Logic has to do with the *creation of form* by the identification of real or abstractable *elements* and the recognition of pertinent *relationships* between such elements. Logic has to do with acknowledging the distinction between *form* and *content*. These are fundamental concepts that clinicians utilize routinely in their work, but perhaps are not aware of them as formal constructs derived from the field of logic.

Scientific thought is based on such principles of logic. It is the recognition of water as being composed of two hydrogen atoms and one oxygen atom that allows us to see water, ice, and steam as different forms of the same thing. It is the understanding of the movement of electrons that allows us to see electricity in its various manifestations as one and the same thing. So, too, physicians recognize that disease has a form independent of its content. Indeed, for the most part physicians do not see the disease itself (and never really see the exact same disease twice), but rather witness various manifestations of it, as symptoms and physical stigmata of disease, which are taken as signs, which they then relate to each other to form a concept of the disease.

The scientific basis of medicine, upon which our effectiveness as clinicians is dependent, is inextricably linked to the application of principles of logic to our observations of disease.

1.7 Symbolic Transformation and Clinical Medicine

There is another conceptual process that physicians employ in their clinical work which sets the stage for and allows the application of logic to clinical problems: *symbolic transformation*. The very term sounds foreign to clinical medicine and might appear far removed from the day-to-day challenges that physicians face in establishing diagnoses and rendering patient care.

When clinicians observe signs of disease, those all-important sense-data that inform the clinician about the presence of a disease, they inevitably use them as symbols *as well as* signs.

There is a marked difference between using symbols as opposed to using signs as tools for processing sense-data. Clinicians invariably treat the sense-data they observe as manifestations of disease both as *signs*, signals to indicate the presence of disease, and *symbols*, items that allow one to think about disease. Indeed, *it is this dual operation of sense-data as sign and symbol together that is the key to realistic thinking about disease* and is at the root of the clinician's practical intelligence.[2] It is the basis of scientific thought.

The next chapter will explore the logical difference between signs and symbols. An awareness of this crucial distinction serves to enhance a physician's understanding of some of the conceptual processes that occur when he or she interviews and examines a patient and seeks to establish a diagnosis.

One feature that sets this new age of medicine apart is that the electronic health record has added another symbolic mode in which to express medical information. The transformation of medical information between verbal, printed, and electronic formats needs to be explored and investigated, for they each carry with them distinctive properties and values. It behooves us as clinicians to understand and elucidate these transformations.

1.8 **Conclusion**

In spite of the evolution of a myriad of functional units among physicians, the opportunities for collaboration among clinicians have never been greater. The ability to access all kinds of information about our patients' medical conditions has markedly improved with the evolution of the electronic medical record. And the ability to communicate efficiently and seemingly effortlessly with other health care providers as well as with patients has been greatly enhanced.

To make the best use of these opportunities and abilities, it is important that clinicians learn to think clearly and coherently about disease and use optimal ways to communicate our practical and direct knowledge of disease to and amongst each other.

Making our communication legible, which is one attribute of the electronic medical record, will not help unless the substance of those communications is coherent and meaningful. The ability to access huge amounts of data about our patients in a wide variety of formats leads to the issue of discrimination, priority, and presentation – which data is most important to have and how is it best shared?

Symbolic logic can help the clinician understand how our clinical concepts are derived, how medical information is structured, and can provide a means for handling the clinical facts that greet us in the workplace, facts which need to be understood in a shared and relatively stable context.

Perhaps this book will motivate some physicians to learn more about symbolic logic and explore in more depth its application to clinical medicine.

REFERENCES:
1. LANGER, SUSANNE K, *An Introduction To Symbolic Logic.* Dover Publications, Inc., New York, third revised edition (1967), pgs. 45-81.
2. LANGER, SUSANNE K, *Philosophy In A New Key.* Harvard University Press, Cambridge, Massachusetts, third edition (1956), pg. 267.

Men occasionally stumble over the truth, but most of them pick themselves up and hurry off as if nothing ever happened.

-*Winston Churchill,* British prime minister

Chapter Two
Signs and Symbols of Disease

2.1 **Sounds and Signs**

A middle-aged woman presents to your office complaining of shortness of breath. This has become progressively worse over the last several months. Recently, when playing with her grandchild, she had to stop and sit to catch her breath.

You examine her and hear a harsh systolic murmur just to the left of the upper sternal border. The remainder of the exam is unremarkable.

You order an echocardiogram that shows an abnormally echo-dense aortic valve with severely thickened leaflets. There is a significant decrease in cusp excursion and the peak instantaneous pressure gradient across the valve during ventricular systole is markedly increased with a measured gradient of 90 millimeters of mercury.

She is referred for further testing and treatment. A surgeon replaces her native aortic valve with a bioprosthetic one.

When you see her in follow-up about eight weeks after her surgery, she states she is feeling well. She is no longer troubled by shortness of breath. She babysits her grandchild three times a week without a problem.

2.2 **The Recognition and Treatment of Disease**

How do we know when a disease exists? How do we distinguish one disease from another? How do we know when a disease has been effectively treated? And how do we communicate our knowledge of disease to others?

14

2.3 **Signs of Disease**

Doctors are trained to recognize signs of disease. A sign is important to the physician because it is interpreted as being a manifestation of a disease process (Figure 2.1).

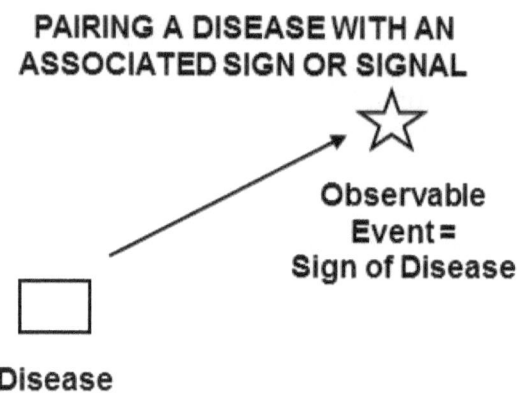

PAIRING A DISEASE WITH AN ASSOCIATED SIGN OR SIGNAL

Observable Event = Sign of Disease

Disease

Figure 2.1

In and of itself, however, a perceptible item which is taken as a sign of disease is meaningless. For instance, the fact that a woman with aortic stenosis has, on examination, a high-pitched sound emanating from her upper chest "means" nothing. It exists as a sensory event – a sound – and might well be ignored.

For a sensory event such as this to be meaningful, the doctor must link this event to something else – the disease process. Indeed, items or elements which we label as signs of disease become significant only to the extent that we can pair them with the disease itself.

However, the mere act of pairing one thing with another is not sufficient to create an entity that is meaningful. That is, pairing a sensory event, such as a heart murmur, with its associated disease is not sufficient to give meaning to that pair.

We frequently deal with pairs of things neither of which can be said to have "meaning." For instance, when eating at a Chinese restaurant, one might ask for a pair of chopsticks. But one cannot say one chopstick or the other has meaning.

Even if we take two dissimilar items and pair them, such the front entrance door to a house and a door bell, which is placed adjacent to it, that act alone does not make one or the other item, in and of itself, meaningful. Another example would be a car and its brake lights. One cannot say that the car itself, or the lights placed at the rear of the vehicle (which light when the car is braking), have meaning. Although the logical relationship between a sign and its indicated object is that of a pair, that relationship of two does not, by itself, create an entity that can be classified as having meaning.

The fact that an item or thing, such as a sensory event (e.g. harsh murmur), takes on meaning arises from the fact that there is a third party – the doctor in the case of a disease and its associated sign – that interprets that item or thing to indicate the presence of something else (e.g. disease). Meaning is a function that involves *three* terms: a perceptible event, which we call a sign, an object, which doctors call the disease, and a subject, which in clinical medicine is frequently either the doctor (or other health care provider) or the patient (Figure 2.2).

THE MEANING OF A SIGN IS A FUNCTION THAT INVOLVES THREE (3) TERMS

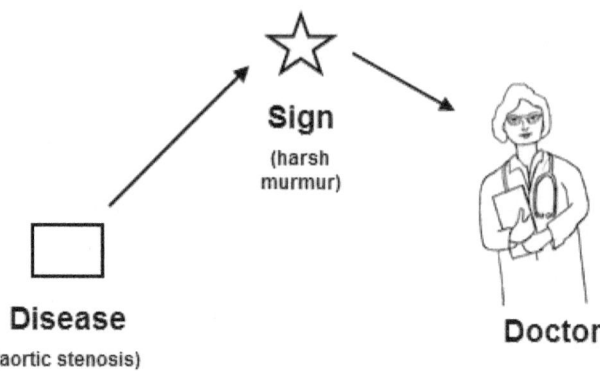

Sign

(harsh
murmur)

Disease

(aortic stenosis)

Doctor

Figure 2.2

In clinical medicine, the meaning of anything that functions as a sign of disease involves these three terms.

Although a disease and its sign are related to form a pair, the doctor finds the sign of the disease accessible and observable while the disease itself exists in the patient in a more complex and perhaps amorphous form (Figure 2.3).

LOOKING FOR SIGNS OF DISEASE

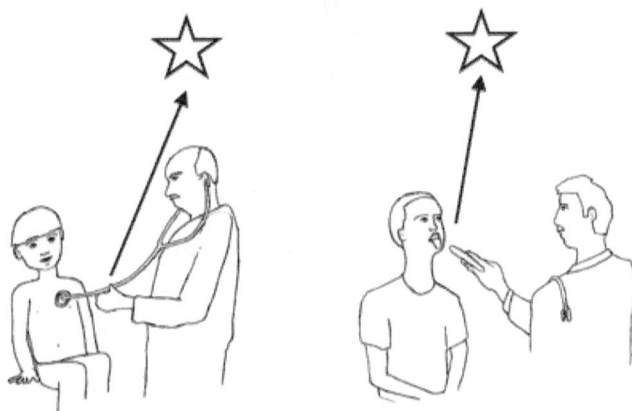

Figure 2.3

The observation of those sense-data which doctors use as signs of disease is the basis for the recognition of disease. As such, we have developed and continue to develop an extensive knowledge of signs of disease and an understanding of the significance of those signs.

If disease did not in some way give off a perceptible signal indicating its presence, neither the doctor nor patient would be aware of its existence.

2.4 When Is A Sign Not A Sign?
A 60-year-old man presents to your office complaining of exertional chest tightness. After performing a history and physical, you decide that the patient may have coronary artery disease and be experiencing angina.

You perform an EKG.

You look for abnormalities that might indicate the presence of coronary artery disease. But there are no ST depressions or T-wave inversions that might indicate the presence of myocardial ischemia. And there are no Q-waves that would indicate the existence of a myocardial infarct.

The EKG is normal.

Undeterred, you order a non-imaging stress test. At one-minute into exercise, the patient develops his typical chest tightness. He is able to exercise four minutes and twenty seconds, stops because of fatigue and dyspnea, and the EKG remains normal throughout the test. Systolic blood pressure, which was 130 mmHg at the start of the test, is 180 mmHg at peak exercise. He reaches 87% of his predicted maximum heart rate.

Despite the absence of any other objective finding, except for the patient's reported symptom of chest tightness during exercise, that might confirm the presence of coronary artery disease, you remain suspicious that the patient has coronary artery disease. He has insulin-dependent diabetes, a family history of premature coronary artery disease in two first-degree relatives, and a markedly abnormal lipid profile.

This is not an uncommon situation in clinical medicine and merits further analysis.

Although physicians are taught to distinguish between *symptoms* and *physical stigmata* of disease, in the realm of logic the patient's subjective symptoms and the objective physical stigmata of disease serve equivalent functions. The subjective complaints given by a patient, which we call symptoms, and the physical stigmata of disease, which are objective and perhaps tangible manifestations of the

19

disease process, are both paired with disease and so serve the logical function of signs. Both the symptoms and physical stigmata of disease are accessible to the doctor, although more often than not it is the disease which is of primary interest to the doctor.

This patient's symptom of exertional chest tightness functions as a sign and is interpreted by the doctor to indicate the presence of coronary artery disease.

But what can we say of the typical EKG abnormalities of coronary artery disease, those objective manifestations of the disease process, such as ST depressions, indicative of the presence of myocardial ischemia or Q waves, indicative of myocardial scar, both of which, in this case, are absent?

First of all, we would be hard pressed to call them signs of disease, in this particular situation and in the strictly logical sense, because they are not present. However, despite their absence, we continue to suspect that the disease process with which they are associated is actually present.

To the extent that the sensitivity of a sign is less than 1 $(S+/D+ < 1)$[1], physicians will always be faced with problems of this nature. And we have developed ways to deal with such problems.

For instance, we categorize signs of disease as true or false. When a sign exists and actually indicates the presence of disease, we classify that sign as a true positive.

In the case of a patient with a disease who does not, for some reason, manifest a sign we typically see associated with that disease, we call the absence of that sign a false negative.

But, if signs of disease are meaningful to the doctor because of their ability to signal to the doctor the presence of disease, it would seem counterintuitive to call the absence of a sign a sign and, worse yet, to qualify this sorry state of affairs by calling it a false negative sign.

In this situation, the sign of disease is not functioning as a sign at all. It is functioning as a symbol[2] (Figure 2.4).

DUAL OPERATION OF SENSE-DATA AS SIGN AND SYMBOL

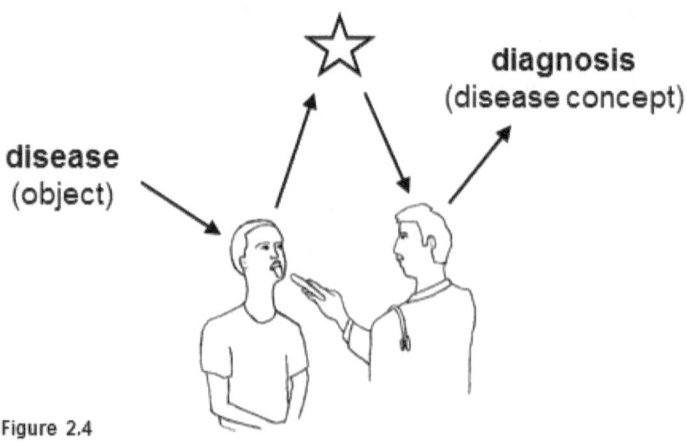

diagnosis
(disease concept)

disease
(object)

Figure 2.4

2.5 The Logical Function of Symbols

We do not talk much about symbols of disease. But we use them quite a bit in clinical medicine.

The distinction between signs and symbols of disease derives from how each function to provide meaning. Meaning, as we have noted, is not an attribute intrinsic to a thing in and of itself. Meaning is not an attribute intrinsic to that item a subject utilizes as a sign. Nor is it intrinsic to an

21

item which is used symbolically. Rather, *meaning* has to do with the *relationships* a subject forms between an item (in this case, the entity which the physician is using as a sign or a symbol) and other things.

The *meaning of a sign* is a function that involves *three* terms: an object (e.g. the disease), the item used as sign, and a subject (e.g. the doctor).

The *meaning of a symbol* is a function that involves *four* terms: an object (e.g. the disease as it exists in nature), the item used as a symbol, a subject (e.g. the doctor), and a fourth term: a concept (e.g. the doctor's idea of the disease) (Figure 2.5).

THE MEANING OF A SYMBOL IS A FUNCTION THAT INVOLVES FOUR (4) TERMS

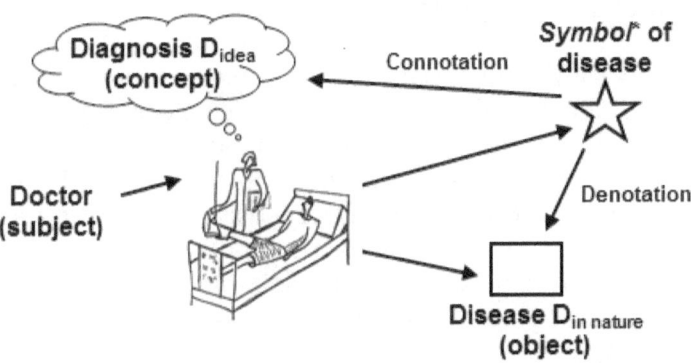

*The *symbol* is being used to represent a sign of disease.
Figure 2.5

A disease actually exists in *two* ways: as *a biological process* that exists in nature and develops in a living thing and also as *a mental picture in the doctor's mind.*

An item, when used purely and exclusively as a *sign* of disease, in a strictly logical sense, *bears no relationship to the disease as it exists in the doctor's mind*. Rather, it is a thing that indicates the presence of a disease in the patient, much as a ringing phone indicates someone is calling.

On the other hand, when that same item is used as a symbol associated with a disease, the subject is using it both to indicate an element in a mental picture or conception of the disease and also to indicate the disease itself as it exists in the patient.

It is important to distinguish between an item we use to signify the presence only of the disease itself, such as a Hemoccult® card that indicates the presence of blood in the stool, and that same object when we use it not only to denote the presence of a disease, but also as a vehicle that allows us to think about the disease and communicate our knowledge of the disease to others.

Doctors for the most part freely navigate this world of signs and symbols without awareness, flip-flopping between using a sign of disease to convey the actual presence of the disease (e.g. "Go see the patient in room 224 – her hemoglobin is 6 and she is hypotensive.") and using a sign strictly in its logical sense, as a symbol, to convey only the thought of it (e.g. "Go check the labs on Mr. Brown and see *if* his hemoglobin has dropped *since* his transfusion yesterday.").

The logical basis of clinical medicine is grounded in this crucial distinction between signs and symbols of disease.

2.6 **Concepts of Disease**

In the clinical example described in section 2.4 of a 60-year-old man presenting with chest tightness, a symptom typical for angina, the dual-operation of that sense-datum as both a sign and symbol leads the doctor to search for other signs of coronary artery disease.

To the patient, his symptom of chest discomfort indicates that there may be something wrong with or in his body, although perhaps he has no idea what that thing is. But to the doctor, the presence of chest discomfort leads to the consideration of coronary artery disease, whether or not that disease actually exists in the patient.

The very fact that the doctor chooses to do an EKG, looking for "ischemic ST-T wave abnormalities," whereas most patients might have no such inclination, tells us that the doctor is reacting to the patient's symptom of chest tightness in a very different manner than the patient himself.

Symbols function in a different way than signs and the kind of meaning a symbol provides is fundamentally distinct from the kind of meaning a sign provides.

As a symbol, the EKG findings identified as "ischemic ST-T wave abnormalities" have the property of *both denotation and connotation*.

The "ischemic ST-T wave abnormalities" function symbolically both to denote and connote coronary artery disease. *Denotation* is the relationship between the symbolic entity "ischemic ST-T wave abnormalities" and the *actual disease* which gives rise to these EKG abnormalities.

The symbolic term "ischemic ST-T wave abnormalities" also functions to connote the *idea* of coronary artery disease.

Connotation is the relationship between the entity "ischemic ST-T wave abnormalities" and the *concept* of coronary artery disease.

When we use the term "ischemic ST-T wave abnormalities" in its symbolic mission of connotation, it does not matter whether or not the disease is actually present. We are using the term to allow us to think about the disease.

It makes perfect sense, when using the term "ischemic ST-T wave abnormalities" in its function as a *symbol*, to consider and talk about the absence of this element as a "false-negative sign" in a patient who, nonetheless, may nonetheless harbor the disease that can give rise to it.

We know that some patients who *do have* a disease (D+) *may not* manifest a particular sign associated with that disease D, and we categorize those patients as having a *false-negative* "sign." Those patients who *do manifest* a particular sign associated with the disease, D, have a *true-positive* sign.

Some patients who *do not have* disease D (i.e. D-) may, nevertheless, *manifest* a "sign" that is sometimes seen in individuals with disease D, and we identify those patients as having a *false-positive* "sign," and distinguish such individuals from the patients who have *true-positive* signs for disease D.

In all these situations, we are treating signs of disease as symbols - as vehicles for thinking about disease.

FOOTNOTE AND REFERENCES:
1. Page 20: S+ = all patients with disease D who manifest sign S of the disease. D+ = all patients with disease D.
2. LANGER, SUSANNE K: *Philosophy In A New Key*. Cambridge, MA: Harvard University Press (1942), *Chapter III: The Logic of Signs and Symbols*, pgs. 53-78.

Everyone wishes to have truth on his side, but not everyone wishes to be on the side of truth.

-*Richard Whately,* logician

Chapter Three
The Disease Process: Its Content and Logical Form

3.1 **Introduction**

Why is it that physicians have no mathematical language in the sense that physicists or chemists do?

If you ask a physicist how much momentum a ball weighing 5 grams would have when rolling due North at 10 mph, she could easily calculate it from a formula incorporating these two terms: the object's mass and velocity. So, too, a chemist, when asked how strong an acid solution is, could tell you by invoking a formula relating the pH of the solution to the concentration of hydrogen atoms in the solution.

But, if you ask a doctor to tell you whether or not a patient had a heart attack, there would be instances in which the doctor would hem and haw. She might ask about the patient's symptoms, or the level of troponin detected at the time the patient presented with his symptoms, and she would want to look at the electrocardiogram. But even then, the doctor might waffle, and answer cryptically: "Maybe."

Physicians understand intuitively, by dealing with living systems on a daily basis, that biology is a very different kind of science than physics or chemistry, although biological systems are made up of matter the behavior of which obeys the "laws" of physics and chemistry. Some may say medicine is "more complicated" or that there are "too many variables" to be easily plugged into a formula that leads to a neat and well-defined answer. So doctors need to talk in terms of "probabilities" and "possible outcomes" and invoke concepts such as "relative risk."

But physicians do approach their work in a systematic and logical manner. What is the framework that forms the logical basis of clinical medicine?

Once it is recognized that symptoms and physical stigmata of disease function not only as *signs* of disease, indicating the *presence* of disease, but also as *symbols*, which allow the physician to *think* about disease, we can begin to understand how physicians create and develop ideas about disease.

3.2 Relationships between Signs of Disease
The primary evidence that a physician has about the existence of disease arises from the recognition of signs of disease. But signs alone are not sufficient to create an understanding of the disease process.

Imagine, for instance, if we listed all the signs of a disease such as lymphoma. This might yield knowledge of the disease sufficient to allow its recognition by the doctor. But can we really say that such a list represents the physician's understanding of lymphoma?

A list of all the signs of lymphoma would not guide the physician to an understanding that would allow appropriate treatment of the lymphoma. Nor would the list bring the physician to an understanding of how to counsel the patient with regard to the disease and its prognosis.

Such a piecemeal list of signs does not bring the physician any closer to an understanding of disease than providing a child with all the letters in a word such as "apple" (i.e. "p, l, e, a") brings the child to an understanding of how to spell the word or, more to the point, an understanding of what the word means.

At least as important to doctors is *what we do with the signs of disease once they are recognized*.

By treating signs of disease as symbolic elements, we can *relate* one to another and create a *logical form* (Figure 3.1).

LOGICAL FORM
The relationships that exist between elements

e R e

e = *element* = sign of disease
R = *relationship between* signs of disease

Figure 3.1

3.3 The Logical Form of Disease

A patient presents to the Emergency Department with fever and malaise. She complains of a cough productive of greenish sputum for the past two weeks. A chest x-ray demonstrates infiltrates in the right middle and upper lobes. The sputum is cultured and grows *staphylococcus aureus*.

The patient is treated with an appropriate antibiotic. She is told she can anticipate a full recovery. Three weeks later she feels well and has resumed all her normal activities.

This patient presents with various signs of disease: malaise, fever, cough, sputum production (which is greenish in color),

29

a chest x-ray showing infiltrates, and the growth of bacteria, *staphylococcus aureus*, from her sputum.

It is the *relations* which we establish between the various signs of disease that provide us with the means to establish the diagnosis, the prognosis, and institute effective treatment.

If we were primarily concerned about the signs of the disease that were most troubling to the patient, we might institute treatment to suppress her cough and fever. But no physician would consider this patient to be effectively treated having suppressed these signs of the disease.

Our *understanding* of the disease is that there exists a bacterial infection in the patient's lungs. And optimally effective treatment is provided by eradicating the infection which, in turn, will lead to the resolution of the fever and the cough.

Our knowledge of disease, therefore, derives not simply from the recognition of signs of disease, but how we put those signs together. This is called the *logical form of the disease* (Figure 3.2).

LOGICAL FORM OF PNEUMONIA

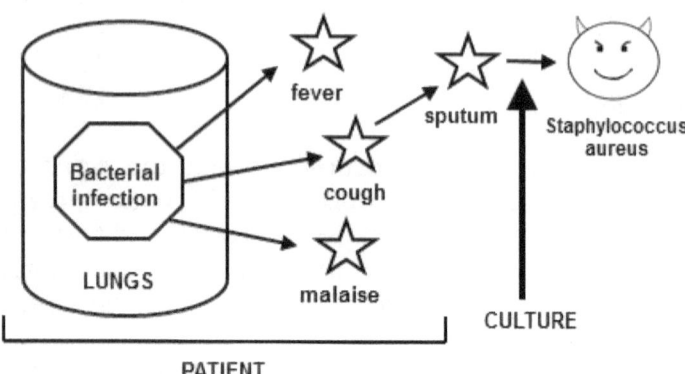

Figure 3.2

The logical form of a disease is a purely abstract formulation. But it is not just any abstract formulation. Doctors do not relate the signs of disease to each other in any manner they choose. The logical form of the disease must mirror the actual disease process as it occurs in nature.

The logical form of an object is an abstract notion that informs us of how that object is "put together." Logical form tells us something about how an object exists or is constructed.

The creation of logical form requires the recognition of real or abstractable elements (Figure 3.3).

LOGICAL FORM
Elements

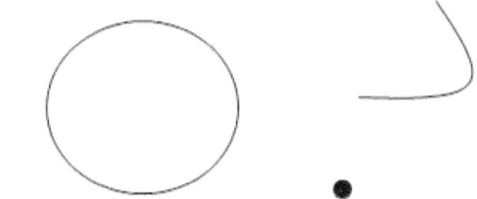

**The creation of logical form requires the
recognition of real or abstractable elements.**

Figure 3.3

The creation of logical form derives from the relationships
we establish between those elements (Figure 3.4).

LOGICAL FORM
Elements and Their Relationships

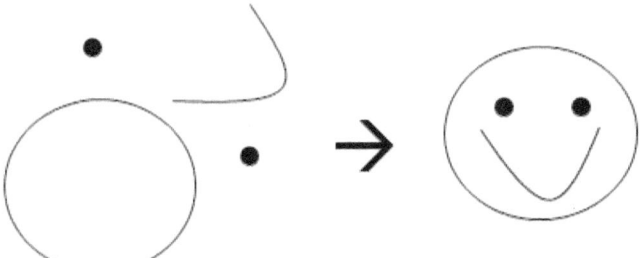

**The creation of logical form derives from the
relationships we establish between elements.**

Figure 3.4

The logical form of an object is an abstract notion that informs us of how that object is "put together" (Figure 3.5).

LOGICAL FORM
Elements and Their Relationships

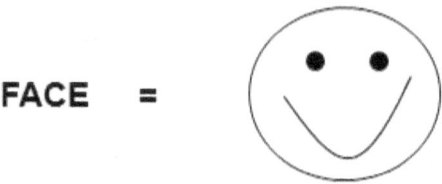

FACE   =

The logical form of an object is an abstract notion that informs us of how that object is "put together"

Figure 3.5

Figures 3.6 thorough 3.12 are examples of different types of logical form.

LOGICAL FORM
Elements and Their Relationships

FACES

Figure 3.6

LOGICAL FORM
Elements and Their Relationships

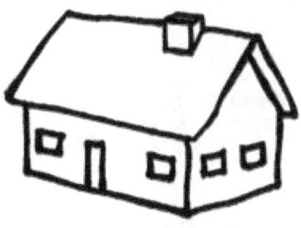

HOUSE

Figure 3.7

34

LOGICAL FORM
Elements and Their Relationships

$$p = mv$$

The linear momentum, p, of an object is equal to the product of its mass and velocity.

Figure 3.8

LOGICAL FORM
Elements and Their Relationships

$$E = mC^2$$

Energy is equal to the mass of an object times the square of the speed of light.

Figure 3.9

LOGICAL FORM
Elements and Their Relationships

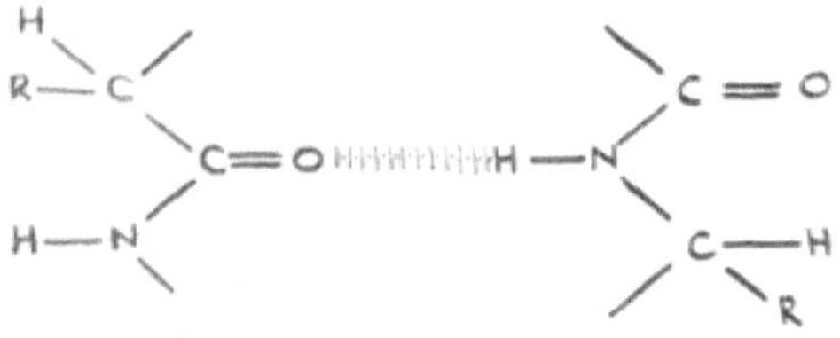

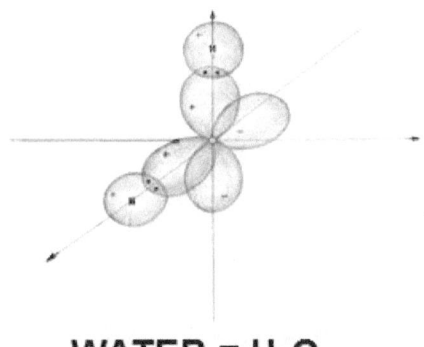

MOLECULAR BONDING

Figure 3.10

LOGICAL FORM
Elements and Their Relationships

WATER = H_2O

Figure 3.11

36

LOGICAL FORM
Elements and Their Relationships

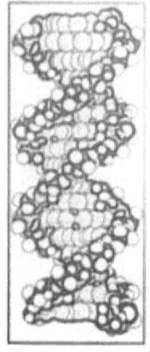 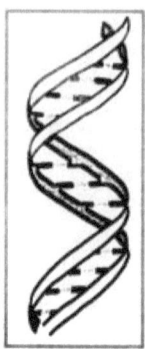

Figure 3.12   **DNA**

3.4 **Establishing a Diagnosis**

There can be no form without making a distinction[1]. The first distinction physicians make is between health and disease. And the first step in making this distinction is the recognition that a sign of disease is present.

Some signs are unique to a single disease. We call such signs "pathognomonic."

If a patient from Connecticut develops a painless, pink, flat, circular rash with a partial central clearing and a "bull's eye" central red area, the physician might recognize this as *erythema chronicum migrans* (also erythema migrans or EM). There exists a disease, and to our knowledge only one disease, that is endemic to Connecticut and manifests this sign.

We call this Lyme disease (Figure 3.13).

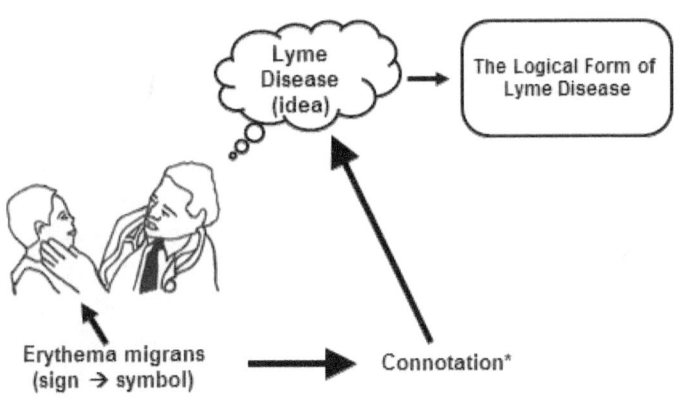

LYME DISEASE

Erythema migrans (sign → symbol)

Lyme Disease (idea)

The Logical Form of Lyme Disease

Connotation*

*See Chapter 2, page 25: *Signs and Symbols of Disease*

Figure 3.13

The logical form of Lyme disease includes, as one of its elements, the sign of erythema migrans. But the logical form of Lyme disease also includes other related elements, symptoms, physical stigmata, laboratory data, and perhaps EKG disturbances, which function as signs-symbols and complete our mental picture of Lyme disease.

If we know nothing more about Lyme disease, other than its association with the pathognomonic sign of erythema migrans, we could go to a textbook of medicine, or perform a search on the Internet and learn more about this disease (Figure 3.14).

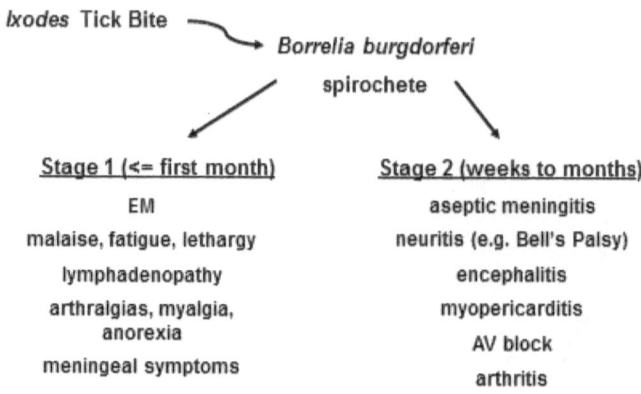

THE LOGICAL FORM OF LYME DISEASE
Elements and Their Relationships

Ixodes Tick Bite

Borrelia burgdorferi
spirochete

Stage 1 (<= first month)

EM

malaise, fatigue, lethargy

lymphadenopathy

arthralgias, myalgia, anorexia

meningeal symptoms

Stage 2 (weeks to months)

aseptic meningitis

neuritis (e.g. Bell's Palsy)

encephalitis

myopericarditis

AV block

arthritis

Figure 3.14

We could learn about the etiology of Lyme disease, its various other manifestations, and could render effective treatment, without having ever treated another patient with the disease.

Thus, by establishing a diagnosis, we identify not only the disease itself as it occurs in nature, but also the logical form of the disease.

The logical form of a disease is the basis for our concept of the disease.

3.5 Diagnosis and the Idea of Class Membership
The logical form of a disease represents a *class* concept.

All patients who manifest signs that fit the logical form of a particular disease may be anticipated to behave in similar ways and respond in a similar manner to intervention.

When we establish a diagnosis, we are taking a sign or signs that indicate the presence of disease, relating it or them as symbolic elements to each other or other symbolic elements, and classifying the patient that manifests those signs and those particular relationships as a member of a particular group.

That patients may be members of diagnostic classes is fundamental to the practice of clinical medicine and a requisite condition that allows for effective treatment.

Having come across a patient with erythema migrans we might establish the diagnosis of Lyme disease based solely on clinical grounds and treat the patient with the appropriate antibiotic.

Should the doctor encounter signs of Lyme disease at a later stage in the process, never observing its characteristic rash during the early phase of the disease, but instead stands witness only to signs that are not pathognomonic of the disease, the physician might confirm the diagnosis by performing serological testing to identify an antibody response in the patient to *B. burgdorferi.*

The diagnosis and treatment of Lyme disease is standardized because, regardless of the stage at which it is recognized or the variable signs which are manifest, physicians agree upon the logical form of Lyme disease and this logical form is the basis of the doctors' concept of the disease.

In this regard, it is important to distinguish between the notion of our *concepts* of disease, that derive from physicians' shared understanding of the logical form of a disease, and a personal and perhaps peculiar *conception* of a disease, which is rooted in an individual's own personal ideas about a disease.

3.6 Different Diseases with Similar Logical Forms

Most signs of disease are not pathognomonic. Different diseases can give rise to the same signs and therefore to distinct logical forms that share the same signs.

Suppose a patient presents with fatigue and is found to have a hematocrit of 21%. The doctor makes the diagnosis of anemia. What is the treatment?

Because many different diseases can cause anemia, a physician would not be able to answer this question precisely based on the information that has been provided.

Although the doctor could order a transfusion of packed red blood cells and bring the hematocrit up to its normal range, this would not be considered ultimately effective treatment.

Within the class of patients with the diagnosis of anemia, there are many subclasses which identify distinct diseases. Effective treatment and prognosis both depend on identification of the specific subclass to which the patient belongs.

The sign of an abnormally low hematocrit is an element in several distinct logical forms, each representing different diseases (Figure 3.15). (For the purposes of clarity and simplicity, not all causes of anemia, such as Vitamin B12 deficiency, are included in this discussion or in Figure 3.15.)

DIFFERENT DISEASES WHICH SHARE THE SAME ELEMENT

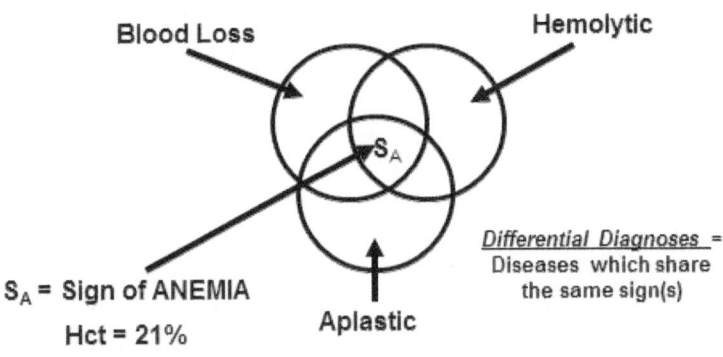

S_A = Sign of ANEMIA

Hct = 21%

Figure 3.15

The doctor must consider the many different logical forms which contain an abnormally low hematocrit as at least one of its elements.

Logical form is a purely abstract notion and is derived from and must manifest in a particular *content*.[2] In clinical medicine, that content is the disease itself.

The process of establishing a list of "differential diagnoses" is our implicit acknowledgment that *different diseases can share the same signs and therefore give rise to logical forms which share the same elements.*

In the case of the patient presenting with fatigue and anemia, we might pursue the evaluation by seeking to determine if there is a problem with blood loss, insufficient production of red blood cells, or both.

With regard to anemia arising from blood loss, we might ask if the red blood cells are being destroyed within the body by hemolysis, or whether there is an exodus of blood from the body, such as gastrointestinal bleeding.

With regard to insufficient production, the doctor might ask whether the source of production, the bone marrow, is no longer functioning normally or whether there is some deficiency, such as lack of iron, which is preventing the normally functioning bone marrow from producing adequate numbers of red blood cells.

The physician would then search for additional signs of disease that could be used to construct a more precise rendering of the logical form of the disease that is present. The doctor's mission is to most precisely align the logical form of the disease with the content of the disease that exists within the patient's body. (Figure 3.16).

DIFFERENT DISEASE CONTENTS WITH SIMILAR FORMS

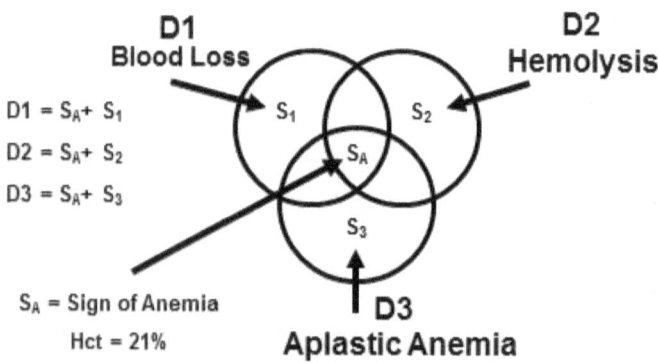

$D1 = S_A + S_1$

$D2 = S_A + S_2$

$D3 = S_A + S_3$

S_A = Sign of Anemia

Hct = 21%

Figure 3.16   *Differential Diagnoses* = Diseases Share Sign(s)

43

The relation between form and content is one of analogy. To establish a diagnosis, the logical form of a disease that we create in our minds must represent most precisely the disease as it occurs in nature.

If the patient is found to have a low serum iron, occult blood in the stool, and an ulcer in the gastric mucosa with signs of bleeding, the doctor would conclude that the patient has an iron-deficiency anemia related to the loss of blood from a bleeding gastric ulcer.

A physician, then, is always working both in the purely abstract realm of the logical form of disease and also trying to identify the content of the disease process that is actually present in the patient.

3.7 The Same Disease with Different Logical Forms

Just as the doctor recognizes that different diseases can give rise to similar logical forms which share the same signs, the doctor also recognizes that the same disease process *can give rise to different instances of that disease, each with somewhat different logical forms.*

For instance, a patient with an acute myocardial infarction due to rupture of a coronary plaque and arterial thrombosis might present with typical or atypical angina, or perhaps no chest pain at all but just shortness of breath, a so-called "ischemic-equivalent." In some instances, the patient with an acute myocardial infarction may present with no symptoms at all, but be found to have, as an incidental finding, an abnormally elevated troponin.

The EKG may show ST elevation, or ST depression, or no change at all in the case of an electrically silent acute infarct.

These differences in appearance may be due to differences in the location of the ruptured plaque in the coronary circulation, or due to differences in the coronary collateral circulation, or perhaps due to a number of other, possibly unknown, factors. These differences in appearances must be reduced to the same pathophysiological event and the patient grouped accordingly, so that timely and effective treatment can be rendered (Figure 3.17).

DIFFERENT FORMS OF THE SAME DISEASE

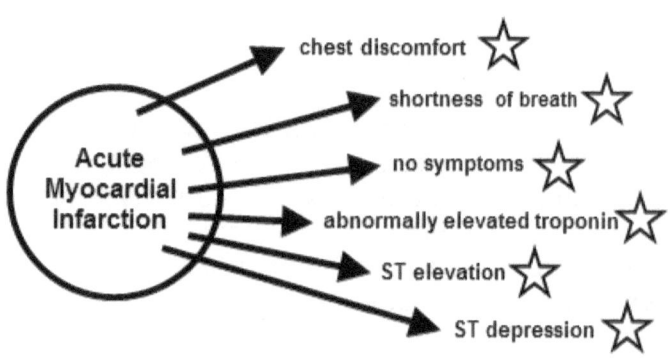

Figure 3.17

3.8 Interpretation and Abstraction

The act of applying concepts of disease to instances of disease as they occur in nature is called *interpretation*.

Much of what medical students learn, in order to become astute clinicians, are the logical forms of the various diseases that have been identified and how to apply these concepts in interpreting the manifestations of diseases as they are observed in clinical practice.

45

They learn how to recognize signs of disease and then, using various diagnostic tests, how to establish whether the disease process that is present fits a particular logical form, thereby establishing (or refuting) a particular diagnosis.

The act of creating concepts of disease based on the observation of its behavior in nature is called *abstraction*.

Medical scientists and clinical researchers study disease to define and articulate its logical form.

3.9 **The Science of Clinical Medicine**
Isaac Newton studied the behavior of objects and developed his basic laws of motion. These are abstract formulae that describe the behavior of the moving objects which Newton observed in nature.

Albert Einstein developed a formula, $E = mC^2$, that describes the relationships between energy, mass, and the speed of light. This is an abstract, logical form that describes a fundamental truth about the behavior of nature.

So, too, the physician doing clinical research studies disease and abstracts its logical form based on what is found in nature. The physician who treats patients with disease does so by interpreting its manifestations in the context of the logical forms so developed.

The physician's "math" lies in the realm of symbolic logic, where signs of a disease are treated as symbolic elements which, in turn, are related one to another to develop the logical form of that disease. A logical form so derived constitutes our concept of that disease.

Clinicians apply such concepts in their work as physicians to establish diagnoses and use their knowledge of diagnoses to provide a broad, relatively stable, conceptual framework to guide their clinical activity, communicate with other health care providers, counsel patients, make treatment decisions, and assess prognosis.

REFERENCES:
1. G. SPENCER-BROWN: *Laws of Form.* New York: E.P. Dutton (1979), pg. 1.
2. LANGER, SUSANNE K: *An Introduction to Symbolic Logic.* New York: Dover Publications; third revised edition (1967), pg. 26.

The truth is so precious and so hard to coax into view – surrounded by its bodyguard of politics and half-truths – that there is simply no time for fuzzy thinking.

-*Andy Grove,* CEO, Intel

Chapter Four
Diagnosis-Driven Medicine

4.1 **Introduction**

The presence of disease is acknowledged when signs of disease are recognized. Those signs can be treated as symbolic elements and related to each other.

The conceptual schemes that arise constitute the logical form of disease. These logical forms are the basis of our concepts of disease. We call them diagnoses.

Disease as it occurs in nature is the content to which such logical forms are applied through a process of analogy.

Clinicians interpret the manifestations of disease which they observe within the context of a vast repertoire of diagnoses.

This conceptual scheme is of enormous practical use to the clinician. To the extent that it guides thought-process, it guides action.

4.2 **Evidence-Based Medicine**

The catch word these days is *evidence-based medicine*. Doctors want to be logical and scientific in their practice of medicine and the ultimate proof of this is to practice evidence-based medicine.

But is it really?

What happens if a doctor is confronted with a clinical situation for which there is no good evidence on which to base one's actions? Is the best course of action to do nothing?

What happens in a clinical situation where there is conflicting evidence? This is not an infrequent occurrence. One might read one study that suggests that a patient with disease X should be treated with A but another study yields the conclusion that a patient with disease X should be treated with B or, worse yet, should not be treated with A. What should the clinician do?

And what happens when the conventional approach, based on the accepted evidence, suggests a particular therapy is effective, but newer, emerging evidence suggests that better therapeutic results might be obtained by instituting a different treatment? When does the clinician go "beyond" the tacitly accepted evidence?

If doctors always acted based only on the existing and accepted evidence, there would be no opportunity to improve treatment and therapeutic results.

If one asked a group of physicians for a show of hands of those who thought it was a good idea *not* to practice evidence-based medicine, it would be highly unusual for any doctor to raise a hand.

But, if you asked the same group of physicians if any of them had ever deviated from the practice of evidence-based medicine for a legitimate reason, the likelihood is that almost every doctor would raise a hand.

4.3 Diagnosis-Driven Medicine

Most physicians practice medicine by grouping patients into diagnostic classes. That is how we think about disease and that is how most of the studies which provide us with our evidence about disease are conducted.

If we are to be logical and scientific in our practice of medicine, doctors should, first and foremost, practice *diagnosis-driven* medicine.

Doctors should identify signs and symptoms of disease, relate them to one another to form a comprehensive list of possible diagnoses, and then focus further clinical activity on establishing the diagnosis, which is to say, identifying the disease which actually exists in the patient (Figure 4.1).

SIGNS OF DISEASE
and their diagnostic constructs

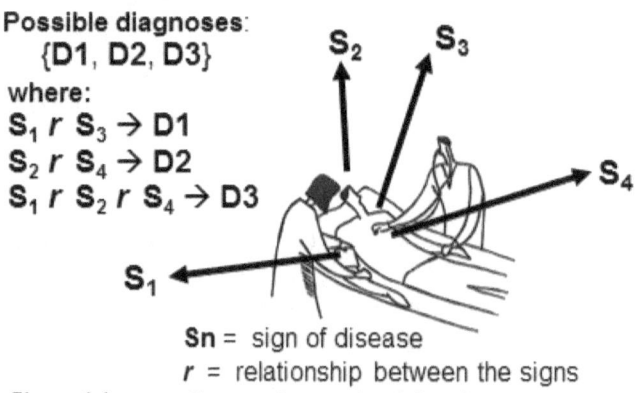

Possible diagnoses:
    {D1, D2, D3}

where:

$S_1 \, r \, S_3 \rightarrow D1$
$S_2 \, r \, S_4 \rightarrow D2$
$S_1 \, r \, S_2 \, r \, S_4 \rightarrow D3$

Sn = sign of disease
r = relationship between the signs
Dn = diagnosis of the disease presumed to be present.

Figure 4.1

It is only after the diagnosis is established that the physician can then ask, "What is the standard of care with regard to the treatment of this disease process?" *The answer to this question will bring the physician to the evidence.*

In doing so, the physician acknowledges that, while a disease process itself usually does not change (although it can – such as in the case of the development of antibiotic resistance), the evidence about that disease, that pathophysiological state indicated by its diagnosis, may well be and often is in a constant state of flux.

51

The initial and primary act in the scientific practice of clinical medicine is to create a relationship between the disease process that exists in the patient and a diagnosis or list of possible diagnoses that fit the logical form of that disease. That is the essence of diagnosis-driven medicine.

4.4 The Significance of Differential Diagnoses

All the diagnostic constructs that pertain to a particular patient together provide the formal context for interpreting the signs of disease which are observed in that patient.

Suppose a patient presents for evaluation of a couple of complaints, S_1 and S_2. Physical exam and laboratory evaluation yield two additional signs of disease, S_3 and S_4. The patient is presented at morning report.

Because of the dual function of symptoms and physical stigmata of disease as both signs and symbols, all the doctors at morning report understand that these observed signs-symbols may, when utilized purely as symbolic elements, be true-positives or false-positives.

One intern suspects the patient has disease D1 based on a relationship he makes between signs S_1 and S_3. Another intern argues that S_1 may be a false finding, and that the relationship between S_2 and S_4 would suggest the presence of another diagnosis, D2. The chief resident presents a case for relating S_1, S_2, and S_4, all of which would support another diagnosis, D3.

A lively discussion follows that may be summarized as follows:

Intern 1: $\mathbf{S_1 \; r \; S_3 \rightarrow D1}$
Intern 2: $\mathbf{S_2 \; r \; S_4 \rightarrow D2}$
Chief Resident: $\mathbf{S_1 \; r \; S_2 \; r \; S_4 \rightarrow D3}$

In this example, S_n = sign of disease, r = relationship between the signs, and D_n = diagnosis of the disease presumed to be present (Figure 4.2).

THE UNIVERSE OF DISCOURSE

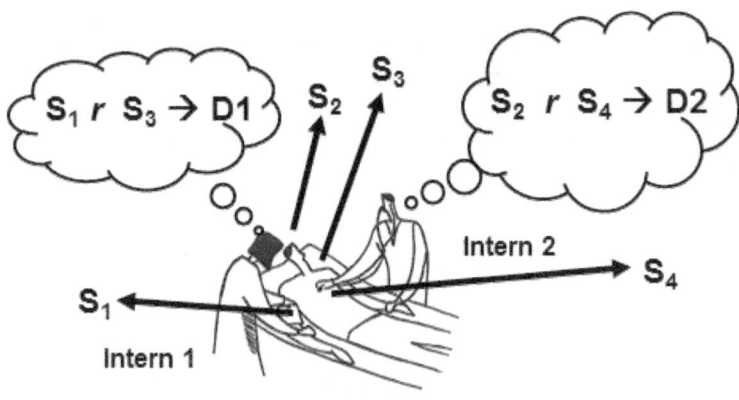

Figure 4.2

Chief Resident: S_1 r S_2 r S_4 → D3

Intern 1 presents the evidence, E1, as it relates to D1 and suggests a test, T1, which would yield the finding of yet another sign, S_5 which, if present, would establish the diagnosis, D1.

In a similar fashion, intern 2 presents evidence E2 and wants to order test T2 to establish the presence (or absence) of S_6 which, if present, would establish the diagnosis, D2.

The chief resident presents evidence E3 which he argues establishes the diagnosis, D3, and wants to start the patient on treatment for this disease right away.

The attending suggests that S_4 might be a false positive finding, and therefore the disease, D3, may not actually be present. She argues the risk of withholding treatment is minimal, and that the diagnosis, D3, could be established as a diagnosis of exclusion if S_5 and S_6 are not present.

Tests T1 and T2 are ordered. Morning report is adjourned with follow-up to be presented later that week.

The differential diagnoses in this case can be summarized as:

DiffDx {*D1, D2, D3*}

and provides, by listing all possible diagnoses, the collection of all the signs of disease and their constituent relations that apply to this particular patient's presentation with this disease.

In clinical medicine, physicians cannot make do with a vague, indefinite, and constantly changing conceptual framework in which to interpret and discuss the signs of disease observed in the patients they treat. Rather, they must make use of recognizable, clearly expressed, and specific concepts which together yield a universe of discourse and provide a formal context for their analysis (Figure 4.3).

THE FORMAL CONTEXT

Differential Diagnoses: {D1, D2, D3}

where

$$S_1 \ r \ S_3 \rightarrow D1$$
$$S_2 \ r \ S_4 \rightarrow D2$$
$$S_1 \ r \ S_2 \ r \ S_4 \rightarrow D3$$

and

$$T1 \rightarrow S_5 \ (?)$$
$$T2 \rightarrow S_6 \ (?)$$

Legend:

Sn = sign of disease

r = relationship between the signs

Dn = diagnosis of the disease presumed to be present

Tn = test that yields a potential sign of disease

Figure 4.3

A list of differential diagnoses forms such a conceptual framework: a universe of discourse; a formal context for analysis. These diagnoses together allow doctors to specify the known and accepted concepts that apply to the interpretation of the signs of disease that are observed in the patient.

Differential diagnoses provide a formal context, which identifies not only the various signs of disease that are relevant to a particular patient's presentation (e.g. signs S_1 through S_6), but also indicates the appropriate and accepted relations that hold between them. And differential diagnoses point doctors to the relevant evidence on which to base evaluation, treatment decisions, and management.

4.5 Clinical Reasoning in the Absence of a Formal Context

A man notices a slight tinge of red in the toilet bowl water after going to the bathroom. This has been going on for several weeks.

He had recently started a new, over-the-counter vitamin. The vitamin was supplied as a large pill in a soft, red capsule. He thought the red color of the toilet bowl water was due to the red vitamin and did not give the matter another thought.

About three months later, he mentioned to his wife that he had noticed some red-tinged toilet bowl water, after having a bowel movement, and volunteered that he had first observed this a few months ago.

The wife told her husband that the red tinge could be blood, as she had a friend who described a similar problem and was found to have bleeding hemorrhoids. She suggested that her husband see a doctor.

This kind of scenario is not uncommon in everyday life. In ordinary thinking the context is usually assumed and not specified. Therefore, individuals may see the same facts, but come to widely divergent opinions about what those facts mean.

In everyday life, the context is frequently indefinite and vague, the elements that enter into ordinary discourse are quite variable, and the relationships between those elements are, more often than not, assumed rather than specified, and not publicly expressed.

In the husband's (personal and individual) conception of the red-tinged toilet bowl water, it was related as an element to a vitamin, consumed orally, which was similar in color. The wife's (personal and individual) conception, based on her own and different experience, related the red-tinged toilet bowl water to blood from hemorrhoids (Figure 4.4).

CLINICAL REASONING IN THE ABSENCE OF A FORMAL CONTEXT

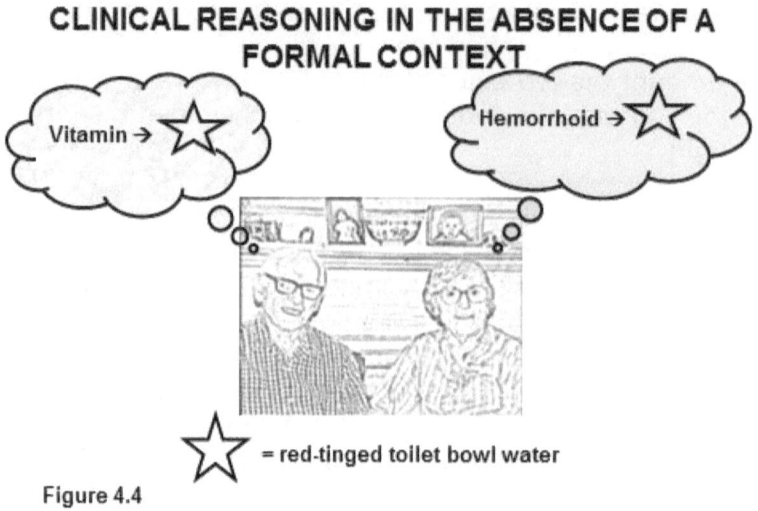

Figure 4.4

Both of these conclusions are logical, although perhaps only one is scientific (and evidence-based).

Logic and science are different but related thought-processes. *Scientific thought is logical, but not all logical thought is scientific.*

Logic is a structured thought-process and arises from the relationships we establish between elements. In any logical discourse, we must specify the elements that belong to the formal context and the relations that may hold between them.

The wife perhaps had no idea that her husband's vitamin was red, and the husband had no idea, perhaps, that hemorrhoids could cause red blood to appear in the toilet bowl water.

So, even though they both were interpreting the significance of the same element, they came to different conclusions because they *failed to agree on the constituent and acceptable relations* between the key element in their discourse and other terms in the "universe of discourse". They failed to agree on the context (Figure 4.5).

UNIVERSE OF DISCOURSE

They *failed to agree on the constituent and acceptable relations* between the key element in their discourse and other terms in the "universe of discourse"

Figure 4.5   = red-tinged toilet bowl water

In science, not only must we agree on the universe of discourse and formal context (e.g. differential diagnoses), but we must insist that the elements that comprise it and the constituent relations bear a semblance to reality.

This is why we practice evidence-based medicine. The evidence ties our thought process and the resultant logical form to reality.

Suppose it is proven that the red capsule that housed the active vitamin, once digested, is no longer red. Then it would be impossible for it to color the toilet bowl water red. That constituent relation would then have no basis in reality and no role in any scientific discourse. The husband's proposition, "Vitamin in red capsule caused the red-tinged toilet bowl water." would not be false; it would be *meaningless*.

The husband was found to have a large malignant colonic polyp which was removed, and he has had no further problems with blood in his stool.

The wife's proposition, "Hemorrhoids caused the red-tinged toilet bowl water," is *false*.

4.6 Differential Diagnoses Guide Physician Action

Constructing an adequate and complete list of differential diagnoses is important to our work as physicians because our concepts of disease guide our activity as physicians.

Suppose a patient presents with an unexplained leukocytosis. The white blood cell count is 30,000/µL.

If the doctor assumes sepsis is present, that diagnostic concept denotes a class of elements and their constituent relations which will guide the doctor's evaluation of the patient. The doctor would seek to establish the presence of certain signs of disease in order to substantiate the diagnosis of sepsis.

He might look for pyuria, or signs of bacteria growing in the blood. He might look for infiltrates on a chest radiograph or symptoms of rigors. He would then try to relate any signs (i.e. elements) of disease observed to each other to determine if he can establish the diagnosis of sepsis -- which is to say, classify the disease which is present within an abstract diagnostic category. If the diagnosis of sepsis mediated by a bacterial infection is established with reasonable certainty, the doctor would then determine the most effective treatment. Is it antibiotic A or antibiotic B?

But, had he considered leukemia as the most likely diagnosis, the doctor would be prompted to look for a different set of elements and their relations to try to prove his hypothesis about the pathophysiological events that led to the development of an elevated white blood cell count.

4.7 **Communication Between Health Care Providers**
When a physician observes a sign of disease, it is transformed effortlessly in the physician's mind into its symbolic equivalent. As a symbolic element, it can enter into a myriad of relationships with other observed signs of disease, from which class concepts emerge and develop, identified under the general headings of diagnoses, and clinical activity is guided by these concepts of disease. But how do we communicate such ideas to others?

The answer: *By externalizing the symbol and presenting it in a form capable of public display.*

Communication is the transfer of information from one place to another. Communication is also shared comprehension. Communication is inextricably linked to the logical basis of clinical medicine. What is being transferred, more often than not, are *symbols* and the *logical form* of disease.

Clinical *information* and *concepts of disease* exist in the physician's mind. There are currently three major modes by which a physician molds a symbolic representation of disease and clinical information for public display: auditory, visual, and electronic.

The physician can express the logical form of disease in a verbal format (talking, dictating), a printed format (written or typed), or enter it into an electronic device where it is frequently expressed in a digital format (Figure 4.6).

THREE SYMBOLIC MODES
Used to store or transfer clinical information from one location to another

- **vMedInfo** = medical information in verbal or auditory format
- **pMedInfo** = medical information in printed or paper format
- **eMedInfo** = medical information in electronic or digital format

Figure 4.6

These modalities offer a means both to store the information and to transmit the information from one place to another.

Each modality offers distinct advantages and disadvantages. And each is distinguished from another in the kind of functions for which it is best suited.

But all share this attribute: they transform the logical form of disease and features of that logical form, as it exists in the physician's mind, into external symbols.

A symbol is a function that involves *four* terms: subject, object, symbol, and *conception*. A sign, on the other hand, is a distinct function that involves only three terms: subject, object, and sign[1].

Verbal, printed, and electronic formats for the storage and transmission of medical information operate in the world of symbols, not signs.

For instance, there could be no electronic medical record if physicians did not transform signs of disease into symbolic elements that are stored digitally in a computer.

The computer may then harbor all the signs of disease that the patient has – an abnormally elevated white blood cell count, an abnormal chest x-ray, and a CT scan showing widespread bony metastases – with one exception: the computer is not sick. The computer stores these signs as symbolic elements. This underscores the crucial distinction between signs of disease and symbols of disease.

When signs of disease undergo symbolic transformation, the resulting symbolic elements function to relate the physician's concept of disease to its content, which is the actual disease process as it exists in reality; but such symbolic elements do not bear the direct relationship to that disease process as do signs, which come into existence by virtue of the fact that the disease process actually gives rise to them.

The black and white image which comprises a CT scan functions as a symbol that allows the physician not only to conceptualize the disease, but also to communicate – that is, transfer information about the disease – from one location to another: from the patient to the computer that stores the CT scan's data elements, from that computer to the physician's mind, from the physician's mind to the medical record, from the medical record to other health care providers, and even back to the patient from which the image originally arose.

The CT scan that shows a mass of neoplastic cells within lung parenchyma as a white spot against a black background, for example, represents a disease (the object) for the doctor (the subject) and simultaneously functions as a vehicle (a symbol) to allow the doctor to think about the disease (conception).

So, too, through the act of speech, a doctor can transfer information about a patient's disease using a concatenation of various sounds, which function as symbols, to other health care providers and the patient. Written and typed words allow a different means of communication of the logical form of disease to other health care providers and the patient.

It is the transformation of a physician's concepts of disease into external and publicly expressed symbolic elements that allows the doctor to communicate his or her knowledge of disease to others.

4.8 Medical Information

The four common ways in which medical information currently can be expressed may be indicated as:

mMedInfo = medical information in the mind of health care provider
vMedinfo = medical information in verbal or auditory format
pMedInfo = medical information in printed or paper format
eMedInfo = medical information in electronic or digital format

Medical information in the mind of the physician is always internal and private unless expressed in a symbolic mode that has the capacity to be made external and public.

Of the other three common symbolic modes in which medical information and the logical form of disease are expressed, they can and do vary in how and to what extent they are expressed externally and publically or held internally and privately.

For instance, medical information in a computer is private and internal but can be made public when expressed on a computer monitor or printed.

Printed medical information, by its very nature, is external and public but may be filed away and made non-public. Such medical information may then be made accessible only to those individuals given rights to view such material.

Dictated medical information makes public the concepts of the disease that the physician holds in his or her mind, but the audible medical information is available only to those who are able to listen to the recorded material. Spoken medical information is available only to those who are able to hear it.

In all these instances, the comprehension of the medical information is predicated upon an adequate articulation of the expressed symbols in a coherent format and the ability of the recipient to interpret and understand them.

4.9 Conclusion

Logic is a structured thought-process[2] and leads to a powerful framework in which to think about disease.

The fundamental act in creating this conceptual framework is the transformation of signs of disease into symbolic elements. This allows physicians to think about disease and communicate ideas about disease to others.

Through the application of principles of logic, physicians create coherent concepts of disease. Formulating such concepts based on accumulated evidence allows the development of a scientific body of knowledge about how disease exists and behaves in the real world and allows for the development of effective treatment strategies.

The second chapter of this book on the logical basis of clinical medicine began by posing a few simple questions.

How do we know when a disease exists?
How do we distinguish one disease from another?
How do we know when a disease has been effectively treated?
How do we communicate our knowledge of disease to others?

To understand the answers to these questions has led to an exploration of the logical function of signs, the distinction between signs and symbols, an analysis of the process of symbolic transformation, acknowledgment of the dual-function of symptoms and physical stigmata of disease as both sign and symbol, the class concept of disease, the role of diagnosis driven-medicine, and the significance of differential diagnoses.

This, in turn, has led to an investigation of the function of evidence-based medicine in building scientific concepts of disease and to the processes involved in the transformation of a physician's ideas about disease into external and public symbolic modes, processes that allow physicians to communicate their ideas about disease to other health care providers and to the patient.

REFERENCES:
1. LANGER, SUSANNE K: *Philosophy In A New Key.* Cambridge, MA: Harvard University Press (1942), *Chapter III: The Logic of Signs and Symbols*, pgs. 53-78.
2. LANGER, SUSANNE K: *An Introduction to Symbolic Logic.* New York: Dover Publications; third revised edition (1967).

Unfortunately, we find systems of education today which have departed so far from the plain truth, that they teach us to be proud of what we know and ashamed of ignorance.

-    G. Spencer-Brown, *mathematician*

EPILOGUE

How to think about disease is one of the most important skills that a physician learns in order to provide effective clinical care.

This book presents an analysis of how a physician transforms perceptions of disease into meaningful information. This is perhaps the primary and fundamental act in clinical medicine.

The quotes which pepper the text of this book center about the concept of truth. Perhaps one of the most important ideas presented herein is the notion that truth is born when the picture of the world in the mind fits most perfectly, by way of analogy, the reality of the world as it presents itself to one's senses and as it is demonstrated to behave.

It behooves the physician, as clinical scientist, to understand the process by which ideas and images of disease are developed and evolve in the human mind, and how it is that the physician can be assured that these ideas and images best fit the reality of disease as it is sensed and observed to behave in the real world. The act of creating the logical form of disease requires that the ideas and images of disease are constructed according to standard rules and principles. The elements and relations that comprise the logical form thus created can be analyzed and tested, through a process of hypothesis and experiment, against reality.

Symbolic logic, therefore, can be utilized to achieve an understanding of disease built of concepts that mirror reality to the extent possible based on current evidence.

Our perceptions of disease constitute an *elemental* understanding of disease: it is a simple truth. The *relationships* that the physician establishes between such elemental perceptions is a much more complicated phenomenon. Those relationships that the physician establishes between the perceptible elements of disease create ideas and images in the physician's mind of the disease that exists in the patient. This kind of truth is distinct and different from elemental truth: it is a delicate truth.

It is by associating such ideas and images of disease, which is to say, its logical form, with the reality of disease as given to us through evidence-based medicine, that the clinician builds a true science of clinical medicine.

The challenges that arise in clinical medicine today frequently expose problems that are in need of solutions. The solutions that need to be found to the problems so exposed are most likely to be most effective when developed by individuals who participate intimately in the practice of clinical medicine on a regular and ongoing basis, frequently day-in and day-out, talking with patients, personally taking care of patients, observing all the results of such interaction as they evolve over time, and observing all the results of any treatment provided, working on the front-lines, so to speak, and privy to all the details that emerge from such activity. In so doing, the clinician develops a justly won appreciation of the realities that face patients and health care providers alike. It is these individuals who are in the best position to define the problems of clinical medicine and set them out in order of priority and importance.

But such an intimate experience with the patient and of disease is not alone a sufficient criterion for success. These individuals must have not only a practical and current knowledge of clinical medicine and disease, but also a facility in analytical tools that allows them to find solutions that work, based on reality; based on truth. Imaginative clinicians, skilled in such analytic tools, will be in the best position to create and offer efficient and effective solutions to the important clinical problems of the day.

Extending the principles of logic to the issues that greet physicians daily in the practice of clinical medicine will allow them not only to be effective clinicians, but will also lead the way to an evolution of clinical medicine that is highly effective in promoting solutions to the problems that face patient and health care provider alike; solutions that are, in the end, true to form.

No great discovery was ever made without a bold guess.

- Isaac Newton, *mathematician and physicist*

The true sign of intelligence is not knowledge, but imagination.

- Albert Einstein, *physicist*

Discoveries of any great moment in mathematics and other disciplines, once they are discovered, are seen to be extremely simple and obvious, and make everybody, including their discoverer, appear foolish for not having discovered them before.

- G. Spencer-Brown, *mathematician*